The Complete Mediterranan CookBook

Delicious Recipes to Improve Your Healthy Lifestyle

Ben Cooper

Table of contents

Marinated Olives with Garlic and Thyme

Prep time cook time: 10 minutes (plus 2 hours to marinate),
Serves: 8

Ingredient:

1/4 cup extra-virgin olive oil

1/4 cup red wine vinegar
3 garlic cloves. minced
2 tablespoons chopped fresh rosemary leaves
1 tablespoon chopped fresh thyme leaves
Zest of 1 lemon
1/2 teaspoon sea salt
2 cups black or green olives drained and rinsed

Directions:

1.In a small bowl whisk the olive oil. vinegar garlic. rosemary. thyme lemon zest and sea salt.

2.Add the olives to your container and pour the marinade over the top. Seal and refrigerate for at least

2 hours. The olives will keep refrigerated for up to 2 weeks.

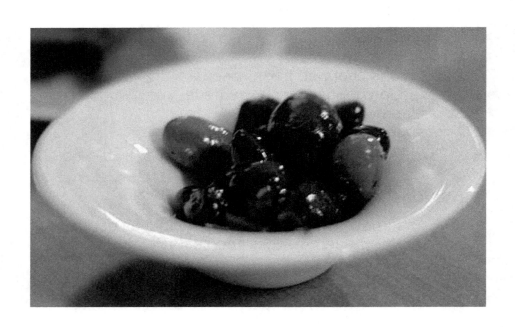

Authentic Tzatziki Sauce

Prep Time Cooktime: 10 minutes (plus 1 hour to chill)
Serve 6

Ingredient:

1 cup unsweetened nonfat plain Greek yogurt
1 cucumber. peeled and grated
1 tablespoon chopped fresh dill
1 garlic clove minced
1/4 teaspoon sea salt
1/8 teaspoon freshly ground black pepper

Directions:

1.Vigorously whisk the yogurt cucumber. dill. garlic sea salt and pepper in a small bowl.

2.Cover well and refrigerate for 1 hour or more before serving.

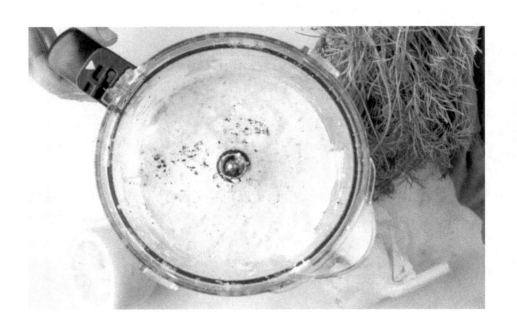

Healthy and Easy Trail Mix

Prep time Cooktime: 10 minutes
Serves: 8

Ingredient:

1/2 cup unsalted roasted cashews
1/2 cup walnut halves
1/2 cup toasted hazelnuts
1/4 cup dried cranberries
1/4 cup dried apricots

Directions:

1.Mix all the ingredient in a bowl. Store in 1/4 cup servings in resealable bags for up to six weeks.

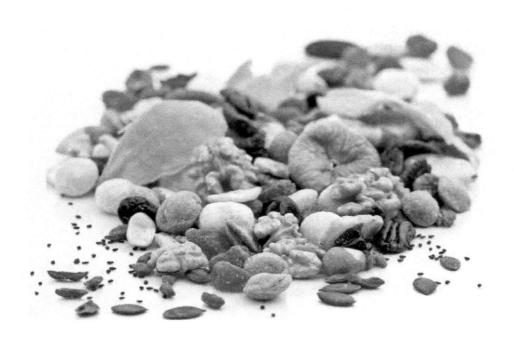

For the Honey-Lemon Syrup:

Preparation time: 10 minutes

Cooking time: 60 minutes

Servings: 4

Ingredients:

¼-cup white sugar

¼-cup water

1-tsp lemon juice

¼-cup honey

Directions:

1.Preheat your oven to 350 °F. Prepare a greased 9" x 9" baking pan. Set aside.

2.Combine and mix the first six Karithopita ingredients in a medium-sized mixing bowl. Mix well until fully incorporated. Transfer the mixture in the mixing bowl of your stand mixer.

3.Pour in the oil, milk, and the egg. Beat the mixture on low speed for 1 minute to a creamy and thick consistency, scraping the mixing bowl's bottom once to avoid lumps.

4.Stir in the chopped walnuts manually using a spatula. Transfer the batter in the prepared baking pan and spread evenly.

5.Place the pan in the preheated oven. Bake for 40 minutes until an inserted toothpick into the center of the walnut cake comes out clean.

6.Let the walnut cake in the pan cool for 30 minutes. In the meantime, prepare the honey lemon syrup.
For the Lemon Honey-Syrup:

7.Stir in the white sugar with water in a saucepan placed over medium heat. Bring the mixture to a boil. Reduce the heat to low, and allow simmering for 5 minutes.

8. Stir in the lemon juice and honey. Remove the saucepan from the heat.

9.By using a knife, make small slashes in a diamond pattern on the top of the cake. Pour the hot syrup over the walnut cake.

Apple Applied Cinnamon Cake Cooked with Olive Oil

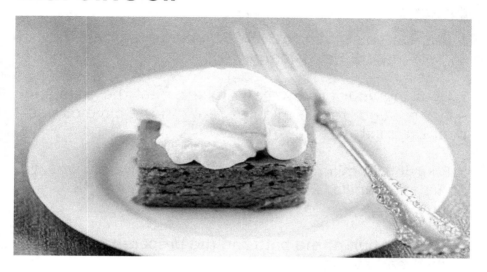

Preparation Time: 20 minutes
Cooking Time: 60 minutes
Servings: 12-slices

Ingredients:

4-eggs
1-cup brown sugar +2-tbsp for apples
1 cup extra-virgin olive oil (as shortening)
1-cup milk
2- tsp baking powder
2½-cups whole-wheat flour
1-tsp vanilla extract
4-pcs apples, peeled, cored, halved, and sliced thinly
1½-tsp ground cinnamon
½-cup walnuts, chopped
½-cup raisins

3- tbsp sesame seeds

Directions:

1.Preheat your oven to 375 °F. Prepare a greased 9" x 9" baking pan. Set aside.

2.By using your electric hand mixer, beat the eggs and a cup of sugar for 10 minutes. Pour in the olive oil and beat the mixture for 3 minutes.

3.Pour in the milk, and add the baking powder, wheat flour, and vanilla. Beat the mixture for another 3 minutes.

4.Transfer half of the batter in the prepared baking pan and spread evenly.

5.Combine and mix the apples, cinnamon, walnuts, raisins, and the 2-tbsp of brown sugar in a mixing bowl. Mix thoroughly until fully combined.

6.Transfer the apple mixture over the batter in the baking pan and spread evenly.

7.Top the apple mixture with the remaining batter. Sprinkle the batter with the sesame seeds.

8.Place the pan in the preheated oven. Bake for 50 minutes until an inserted toothpick into the center of the apple-cinnamon cake comes out clean.

Naturally Nutty & Buttery Banana Bowl

Preparation Time: 5 minutes
Cooking Time: 0 minutes
Servings: 4
Serving Size: 1-cup

Ingredients:

4- cups vanilla Greek yogurt
2-pcs medium-sized bananas, sliced
¼-cup creamy and natural peanut butter
1-tsp ground nutmeg
¼-cup flaxseed meal

Directions:

1.Divide the yogurt equally between four serving bowls. Top each yogurt bowl with the banana slices.

2.Place the peanut butter in a microwave-safe bowl. Melt the peanut butter in your microwave for 40 seconds. Drizzle one tablespoon of the melted peanut butter over the bananas for each bowl.

3.To serve, sprinkle over with the ground nutmeg and flax-seed meal.

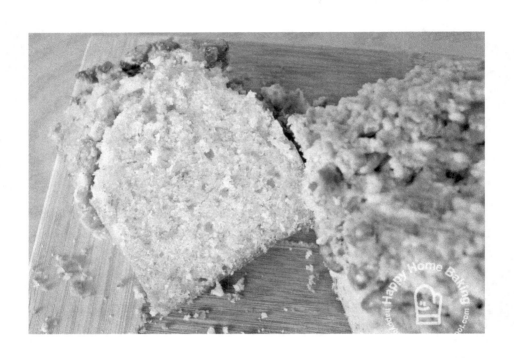

Queenly Quinoa Choco Crunch Baked Bars

Preparation Time: 5 minutes
Cooking Time: 20 minutes
Servings: 10
Serving Size: 2-square bars

Ingredients:

2½-tbsp peanut butter with roasted peanuts
2-tbsp water
1-lb. semi-sweet chocolate bars, chopped into small pieces
1-cup dry quinoa
½-tsp vanilla
1-tbsp natural peanut butter

Directions:

1.Preheat for 10 minutes a heavy-bottomed pot placed over medium-high heat.

2.Meanwhile, prepare a baking sheet lined with parchment paper. Set aside.

3.Make a peanut butter drizzle by stirring the peanut butter with roasted peanuts with water in a small mixing bowl until fully incorporated. Set aside.

4.Add the quinoa by batch, ¼-cup at a time to pop. Allow each batch to sit at the bottom of the pot, stirring occasionally. Once the quinoa starts to pop, swirl it constantly for 1 minute until the popping subsides.

19

(This can happen too quickly, so ensure to take it off lest the quinoa turns brown.) Set aside.

5.Place the chopped chocolate bars in a microwave-safe mixing bowl. Melt it in your microwave for 30 seconds.

6.Add the popped quinoa, vanilla, and peanut butter in the mixing bowl of the melted chocolate. Mix thoroughly until fully combined.

7Transfer the chocolate-quinoa mixture in the prepared baking sheet. You need not spread the mixture across the sheet; else, it gets too thin. Simply form a roughly square shape of the mixture, about half an inch thick, in the middle of the sheet.

8Pour the peanut butter drizzle over chocolate-quinoa square. By using a spatula, spread gently the drizzle entirely around the square.

9.Refrigerate the mixture for an hour until it becomes completely a firm cake. To serve, slice the cake into small square bars.

Phyllo Pastry Balkan Baklava

Preparation Time: 30 minutes
Cooking Time: 35 minutes
Servings: 18
Serving Size: 1-slice

Ingredients:

For the Baklava:

12-sheets phyllo pastry dough 1-tsp ground cloves
2-tsp ground cinnamon 2-cups walnuts, chopped 1-cup sesame seeds
2-cups almonds, chopped 3-tbsp honey
1-cup extra-virgin olive oil (for brushing the dough)
18-pcs whole cloves (1 for each piece of baklava slice)

Directions:

For the Baklava:
1.Preheat your oven to 350 °F.

2.Mix the ground cloves, cinnamon, walnuts, sesame seeds and almonds with honey in a mixing bowl.

3.Brush with olive oil 4-sheets of phyllo pastry, on both sides of each. Lay the oiled sheets on top of each other in a 9" x 9" baking pan.

4.Transfer half of the nut mixture on top of the oiled sheets and spread evenly.

5.Brush with olive oil another set of 4-sheets of phyllo pastry, on both sides. Lay this set of oiled sheets over the nut mixture.

6.Empty the mixing bowl with the remaining nut mixture over the oiled sheets and spread evenly. Top the nut mixture with the last set of 4-sheets of phyllo pastry, brushed in the same manner as the other previous sets.

7.Slice the baklava into 18-equally sized pieces. Top each slice with one whole clove.

8.Place the baking pan in the preheated oven. Bake for 35 minutes until the top turns golden brown. Prepare for the honey syrup while the baklava is baking.

For the Honey Syrup:

Ingredients:

1-pc lemon, rind
1-cinnamon stick
2-cups sugar
1-cup honey 2-cups water
2- pc lemon, juice

Directions:

1.Combine the lemon peel, cinnamon stick, and sugar with honey and water in a saucepan placed over medium heat. Bring the mixture to a boil. Reduce the heat to low, and simmer for 15 minutes.

2.Let the syrup to cool down before stirring in the lemon juice.

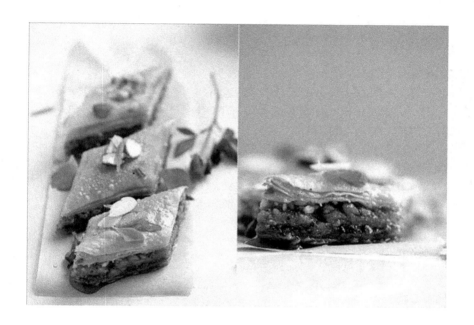

Baked Apple Delight

Preparation Time: 10 minutes
Cooking Time: 1 hour
Servings: 6

Ingredients:

6 Apples
3 Tablespoons Almonds, Chopped
1/3 Cup Cherries, Dried & Chopped Coarsely
1 Tablespoon Wheat Germ
1 Tablespoon Brown Sugar
¼ Cup Water
½ Cup Apple Juice
1/8 Teaspoon Nutmeg
½ Teaspoon Cinnamon
2 Tablespoons Dark Honey, Raw
2 Teaspoons Walnut Oil

Directions:

1.Start by heating your oven to 350, and then blend your almonds, wheat germ, brown sugar, cherries, nutmeg and cinnamon in a bowl. Set this bowl to the side.

2.Core your apples starting from their stem, and chop into ¾ inch pieces. Place this mixture into each hole. Arrange the apples upright in a baking dish. A small one will work best. Pour in your apple juice and water, and then drizzle the oil and honey over top.

3.Cover with foil, and cook for fifty to sixty minutes. The apples should be tender.

4.Serve at room temperature or immediately.

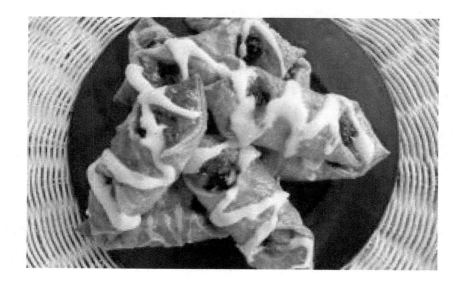

Crepes with passion fruit

Preparation time: 5 minutes

Cooking time: 10 minutes

Servings: 4

Ingredients:

Crepes Sauce
Two eggs
1/25 cups oat milk 1 cup flour
1/5 tbsp butter
½ cup of sugar
¾ cup of passion fruit

Directions:

1.Mix eggs, milk, and flour and keep it aside.

2.Mix sugar with passion fruit and boil it to reduce the concentration to half.

3.Melt the butter and spread crepe mixture in a pan and cook for 2 minutes from both sides.

4.Transfer the crepe to a plate with sauce and serve.

Fennel and seared scallop's salad

Preparation time: 30 minutes
Cooking time: 10 minutes
Servings: 4

Ingredients:

1grapefruit 1 tbsp olive oil
1 tsp raw honey
1/2 tsp chopped fennel seeds
1/4 tsp sea salt
Pinch of black pepper
12 sea scallops
1/2 sliced
3 cups torn red leaf lettuce
12 toasted almonds

DIRECTIONS

1.Strain the grapefruit juice in a cup

2.For the dressing: Transfer juice into a small bowl & whisk oil, add water, honey, fennel, salt & black pepper.

3.Set it aside.

4.Season scallops with remaining fennel & remaining salt.

5.Heat skillet & brush with remaining oil. Cook scallops for five minutes, flipping halfway, till they become lightly from both sides. Transfer it to a plate & cover it.

6.Repeat the same with remaining.

7.Set aside the dressing. In a bowl, toss the fennel & lettuce with the remaining dressing. Divide the fennel salad among the serving plates. Top each salad with the grapefruit pieces & cooked scallops.

8.Drizzle the reserved dressing over scallops & top with the almonds.

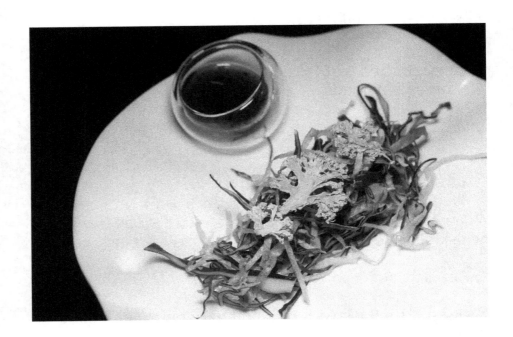

Fruity asparagus quinoa salad

Preparation time: 15 minutes
Cooking time: 5 minutes
Servings: 7

Ingredients:

2 cups cooked quinoa
3 tsp olive oil
30 sliced spears asparagus
1/2 tsp salt
1/4 tsp pepper Two cloves garlic
Salt and pepper
16 sliced strawberries
4.5 oz mozzarella cheese
1/3 cup Balsamic Vinaigrette
2 tbsp basil

Directions:

1.Place cooked quinoa in a bowl.

2.Prepare the balsamic vinaigrette & set aside.

3.Heat olive oil in a pan to overheat.

4.Once heated, add asparagus & garlic.

5.Sprinkle with salt & pepper. Cook 2-3 min.

6.Add asparagus to quinoa.

7.Mix the strawberries, balsamic vinaigrette & cheese.

8.Toss to mix well. Top salad with the basil.

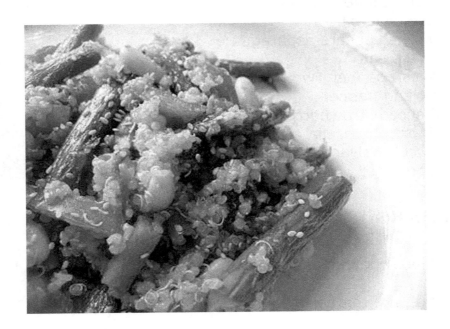

Easy Apricot Biscotti

Preparation Time: 20 minutes
Cooking Time: 50 minutes
Servings: 24

Ingredients:

2 Tablespoon Olive Oil
¼ Cup Almonds, Chopped Course
¾ Cup Whole Wheat Flour
½ Teaspoon Almond Extract, Pure
2/3 Cup Dried Apricots, Chopped
2 Tablespoons Dark Honey, Raw
2 Eggs, Lightly Beaten
1 Teaspoon Baking Powder
¼ Cup Brown Sugar
2 Tablespoons Milk, 1%
¾ Cup All Purpose Flour

Directions:

1.Preheat your stove to 350, and then get out a bowl. Whisk your all-purpose whole wheat flour and baking powder together.

2.Add in your milk, honey, canola oil, eggs and almond extract together. Stir until it become a dough like consistency and then add in your almonds and apricots.

3.Place flours on your hands and then mix everything. Place your dough on a cookie sheet and flatten it to be about a foot long and three inches wide. It should be about an inch tall.

4.Bake for twenty-five to thirty minutes. It should be light brown.
Take it out and allow it to cool for ten to fifteen minutes. Cut into twenty- four slices by cutting crosswise.

5.Arrange the cut slices face down on the baking sheet, baking for another fifteen to twenty minutes. It should be crisp, and allow it to cool before serving.

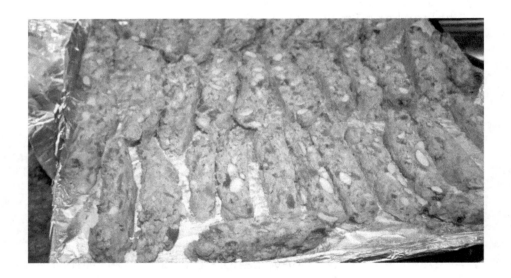

Garden salad with orange and olive

Preparation time: 15 minutes
Cooking time: 0 minute
Servings: 4

Ingredients:
5 oranges
4 cups rocket spinach
150 g feta
1 cup olives
2 tbsp olive oil
A pinch of salt
1 clove garlic

Directions:

1.Peel & dice 4 of the oranges

2.Combine oranges, olives & leaves in a bowl.

3.Crumble feta over the top of the salad.

4.Whisk together the final orange juice, olive oil, salt, and as much garlic as you like. Taste & adjust seasoning according to requirement.

5.Pour dressing on the salad & toss gently to mix well.

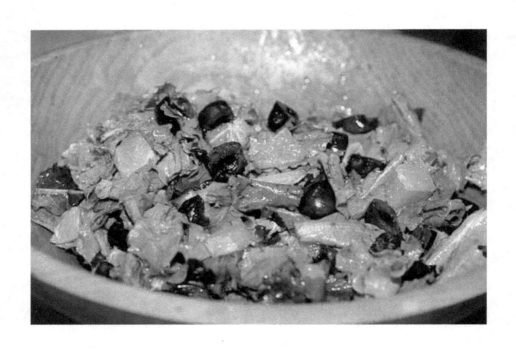

Chickpea Sunflower Sandwich

Preparation time: 20 minutes
Cooking time: 0 minute
Servings: 4

Ingredients:

Garlic Herb Sauce
1 tbsp Lemon juice
¼ cup Prepared hummus
2 tbsp dill
Water as needed
2 minced Garlic cloves Chickpea Sunflower Sandwich
1 tbsp Maple syrup
¼ cup Sunflower seeds roasted
15 oz chickpeas
3 tbsp Mayonnaise
1/2 tsp Dijon or spicy mustard Pepper to taste
¼ chopped Red onion Eight slices of wheat bread
2 tbsp dill
Optional Toppings
Lettuce
Sliced avocado Tomato
Onion

DIRECTIONS

1.To prepare the sauce (garlic herb): mix minced garlic, dill, lemon, and hummus in a bowl. Now set aside.

2.In another bowl, mash the chickpeas roughly. To add texture, leave some in large chunks. Then add vegan mayo or tahini, sunflower seeds, maple syrup, mustard, chopped dill, pepper, and red onion. Mix them.

3.Toast bread in vegan oil or butter (optional).

4.Take four slices of bread. Scoop your sunflower seed filling and chickpeas on them. Add the garlic herb sauce along with your optional toppings. Top with the more four slices of bread to form a sandwich.

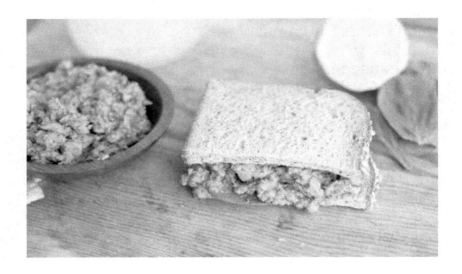

Balsamic Vinaigrette

Preparation time: 4 minutes
Cooking time: 0 minute
Servings: 4

Ingredients:

¼ cup Balsamic vinegar
1 tbsp Dijon mustard
2 tbsp Honey
¾ cup Canola Oil One Garlic clove
½ tsp black pepper
1 tsp Poppyseed

Directions:

1.Take a food processor and blend all ingredients in it for 3-4 minutes, thoroughly emulsified. (You can also take a jar and shake all the ingredients vigorously in it, as an alternative)

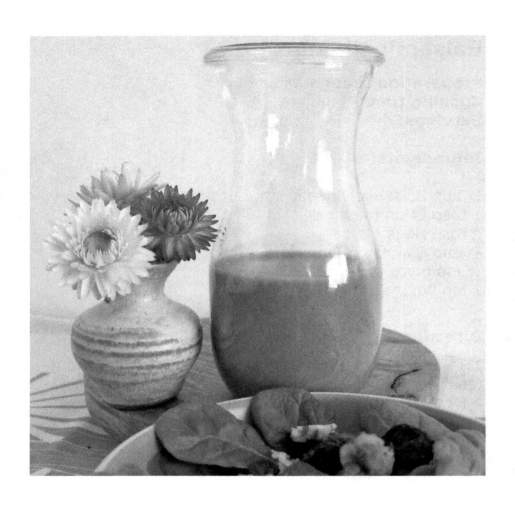

Easy Chia Seed Pudding

Preparation time: 5 minutes
Cooking time: 0 minute
Servings: 4

Ingredients:

½ cup Chia Seeds
1.5 cup of rice milk
1 tsp Vanilla Extract
¼ tsp Cinnamon
¼ cup Maple Syrup

Directions:

1.Take a bowl or a mason jar, add the chia seeds, maple syrup, vanilla, rice milk, and cinnamon. Mix well!

2.Make sure chia seeds do not stick to container sides. Cover the mixture and refrigerate (at least 4 hours or even overnight).

3.You can also add fruit (optional) before serving.

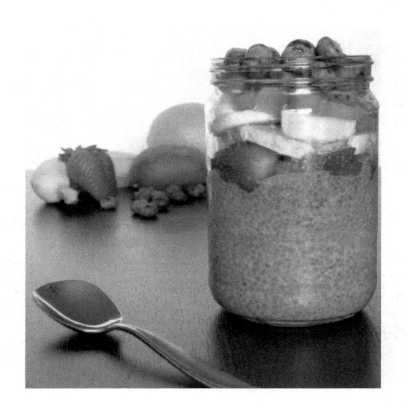

Herb Pesto

Preparation time: 5 minutes
Cooking time: 0 minute
Servings: 4-5

Ingredients:

½ cup Parsley leaves
1 cup basil leaves
2 Garlic cloves
½ cup Oregano leaves
2 tbsp lemon juice
¼ cup Olive oil

Directions:

1.Put the garlic, basil, oregano, and parsley in a food processor; pulse (for 3 minutes until finely chopped).

2.Form a thick paste by Drizzling the olive oil on the pesto. Scrape down the sides as well.

3.Add the pulse and lemon juice; Blend.

4.Take a sealed container and store the pesto in it; Refrigerate (for one week).

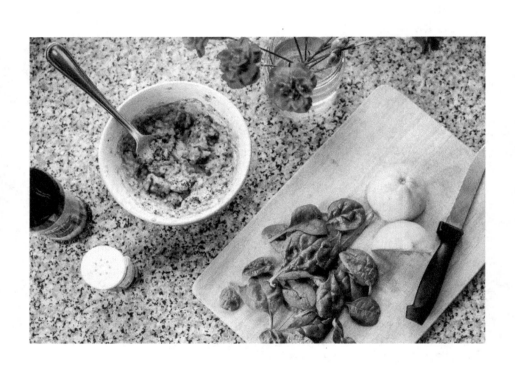

Smoothie Bowl

Preparation time: 4 minutes
Cooking time: 0 minute
Servings: 1

Ingredients:

1 tbsp shredded coconut
¾ cup blueberries
1 tsp Honey
½ sliced banana
3 tbsp plain coconut milk
1 tbsp Blueberries
½ cup of Organic and Frozen strawberries
½ cup Water

Directions:

1.Combine all the smoothie bowl ingredients (except coconut and fresh berries) in a high-speed blender.

2.Allow all the ingredients to be like a creamy sorbet; blend.

3.Pour the mixture into a bowl

4.Garnish the smoothie with coconut and fresh berries. Eat!

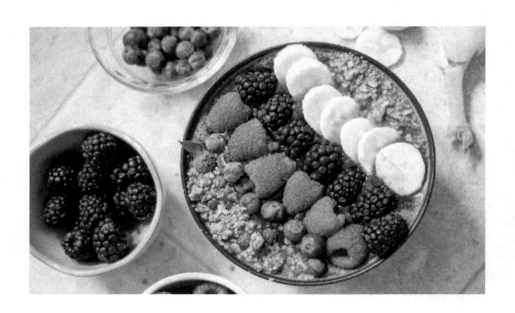

Irish Colcannon

Preparation time: 5 minutes
Cooking time: 30 minutes
Servings: 6

Ingredients:

85 g Russet potato Three Parsnips
1.5 cup Green peas
1 cup Green cabbage
1 diced Onion
1 cup chopped Kale
3 tbsp Olive oil
Black pepper to taste
2 minced Garlic cloves Sea salt

Directions:

1.Place potato and parsnips in a pot of water (large) and bring the ingredients to a boil. Cook until tender (over high heat) for about fifteen minutes.

2.Use a sieve to remove the cooked vegetables. Do not drain the remaining cooking liquid left in the pot; reserve for later.

3.Take a shallow bowl, and with 1/3 cup of the cooking liquid and 2 tbsp. Of the olive oil, mash the vegetables in it. Keep adding as much
cooking liquid as required to remove the lumps. You can also use a hand blender.

4.Layout mashed parsnip mixture on a foil-covered plate.

5.Now, add chopped kale and shredded cabbage to the parsnip water. Cook until the cabbage is just slack (for a few minutes).

6.For this step, drain the kale and cabbage thoroughly and return them to the pot. Cover.

7.Take a skillet (large) and heat 1 tbsp of olive oil in it using medium heat. Add and cook the chopped garlic and onion until it softens.

8.Further, also add the cooked garlic and onions to the pot with the greens and cabbage. Now also add the peas.

9.In the middle of an empty serving bowl, place the parsnip and potato mash. Add and mix the cooked vegetables in. Season with salt and pepper. Serve! (As lunch or as a side dish).

Vegan Banana Bread

Preparation time: 5 minutes
Cooking time: 60 minutes
Servings: 12

Ingredients:

1/3 cup Vegetable oil
2 tbsp Agave nectar
1/8 tsp Salt
1.5 cup Whole wheat flour
½ cup Applesauce
1 tsp Baking soda Four Bananas
1.5 tsp Vanilla extract
½ Sugar
4 tbsp Flax seeds

 Directions:

1.Preheat the oven to 350°F.

2.Firstly, peel the bananas and then mash the peeled bananas with a fork. Place the mashed bananas in a mixing bowl.

3.Now, take a wooden spoon and mix the mashed bananas with vegetable oil using it.

4.Add sugar, applesauce, salt, vanilla, baking soda, agave nectar, and ground flaxseeds in the bowl; stir.

5.Add flour and Stir thoroughly. Pour the mixture into a 9 x 5 x 3-inch loaf pan (greased).

6.Bake for a good 50-60 minutes, until the (top) springs back become slightly depressed. Cool and serve!

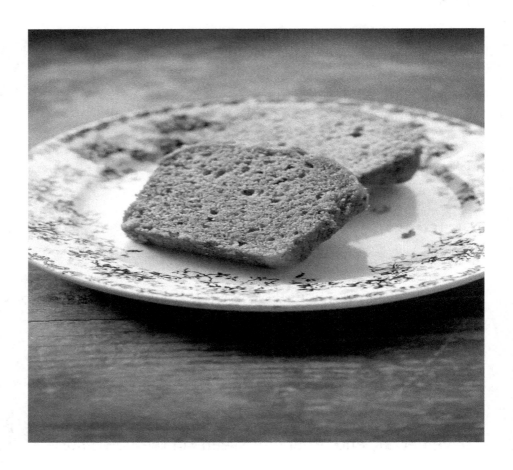

Vegetable Broth

Preparation time: 10 minutes
Cooking time: 60 minutes
Servings: 2

Ingredients:

2 cups Sliced celery stalks
2 tbsp Olive oil
Four chopped carrots
2 chopped onions
½ tsp Dried thyme
8 cups Water
¼ cup Italian parsley
2 Bay leaves
4 Garlic cloves
1 tsp Black peppercorns

Directions:

1. Take a large saucepan, and heat oil in it over medium heat. Add garlic, celery, carrots, and onions. Cook and stir (occasionally) for about 5 minutes.

2. Add peppercorns, water, thyme, parsley, and bay leaves. Set the heat to high now. Bring it to a boil. Now stir again while also reducing heat to medium-low.

3. Let the mixture simmer for about an hour, uncovered.

4. Take a fine-mesh strainer and place it over a large pot. Pour all contents into the strainer. Reserve the broth while discarding the solids.

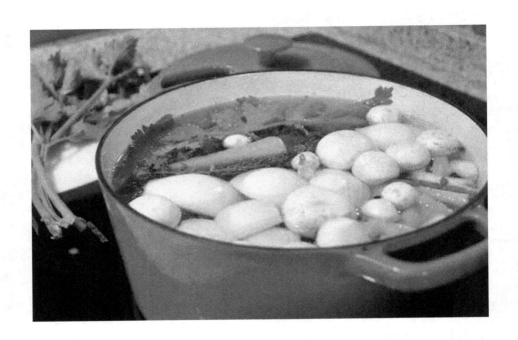

Festive Cranberry Stuffing

Preparation time: 5 minutes
Cooking time: 30 minutes
Servings: 4

Ingredients:
1 cup diced tart apples
¼ tsp Poultry seasoning
3 cups Soft bread
2 tbsp butter
¼ cup Apple juice
¼ cup chopped celery
½ cup diced cranberries

Directions:

1.Preheat the oven to 350°F.

2.Take a large bowl. In it, combine all ingredients; toss and mix.

3.Take a casserole dish (lightly greased). Place the mixture in it and Bake for 30 minutes.

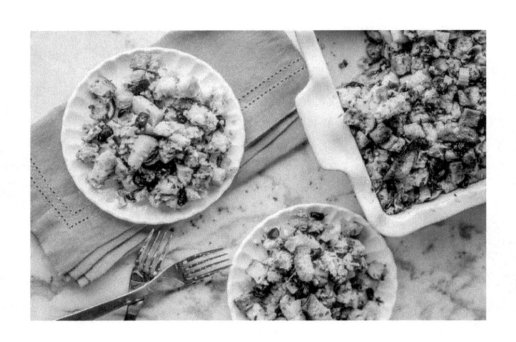

Simple Puerto Rican Sofrito

Preparation time: 5 minutes
Cooking time: 0 minute
Servings: 24

Ingredients:
Chopped Spanish onion
1 tsp salt
5 Stemmed aji dulce peppers
1 bunch Cilantro
1 Chopped green pepper
10 Garlic cloves

Directions:

1.Wash all the ingredients thoroughly before using.

2.Take a blender. Add onions first, and then add all the other ingredients (in small batches).

3.To use within a week, you will be required to refrigerate a portion of your sofrito (in an airtight container. To use within four months or so, freeze in in an ice cube tray or small containers. It is not required to thaw before cooking.

4.Add 2 tbsp. Of sofrito if and whenever you make rice, soups, beans, and stews!

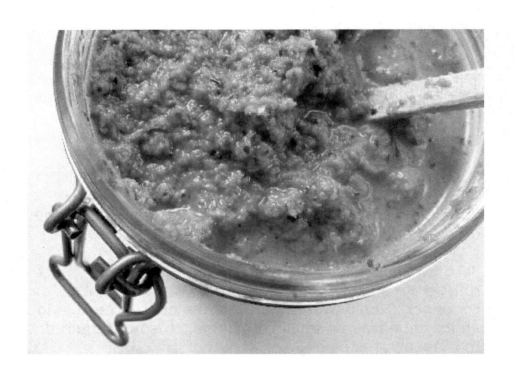

Vegetable Curry

Preparation time: 30 minutes
Cooking time: 30 minutes
Servings: 5

Ingredients:

1 tsp Fennel seeds
1 tsp Cumin seeds
1 tbsp Coconut oil
2 cups Basmati rice
1 tsp Coriander seeds
1 tsp Mustard seeds
1 tsp Hot chili flakes
¼ tsp Black peppercorns
1 grated ginger
1 chopped Onion
1 tsp Turmeric
1 Chopped Carrot
6 oz Coconut milk
1.5 cups chopped Cauliflower
1 cup Green peas

Direction:

1.Take a cast-iron skillet, and add dry spices to it. Heat (low-medium heat) for 2 minutes.

2.Cook the rice while the spices are heating up. (As per theon the package).

3.Add coconut oil and sauté for about 2-3 minutes (low-medium heat). Heat until the spices start popping and turn brownish.

4.Add ginger, hot chili flakes, and turmeric. Cook (low-medium heat) until aromatic for about six minutes.

5.Remove from heat make a paste of the cooked spices by blending them with the onion.

6.Take a separate pan, and heat the coconut milk in it until it starts to bubble up. Add the spice paste; whisk.

7.Add all the vegetables and for 10 minutes, let them simmer until tender.

8.Serve over rice (as per need) and enjoy!

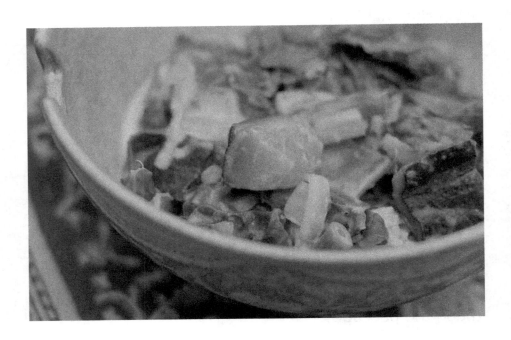

Tabbouleh

Preparation time: 30 minutes
Cooking time: 0 minute
Servings: 4

Ingredients:

1 cup bulgur
1 cup sliced Cucumbers
1 cup sliced Radish
4 sliced scallions
1 bunch of Chopped mint leaves
2 tbsp lemon juice
½ cup olive oil
Pepper to taste Kosher salt to taste

Directions:

1.Fill a large bowl halfway with hot tap water and stir bulgur into it for 20 to 30 minutes. Let it absorb water enough to not be mushy but soft.

2.In a large bowl, put mint and the vegetables sliced earlier.

3.Drain excess water off the bulgur by squeezing, one at a time. Squeeze tightly by holding it over a sink or a sieve, adding each bulgur squeezed into the vegetable bowl.

4.Add olive oil and lemon juice into the salad. Blend all the ingredients by using either a large spoon or hands. Add salt and pepper with seasoning to taste (if desired).

5.Serve it as a side dish for dinner or with crusty bread as a lunch. Enjoy!

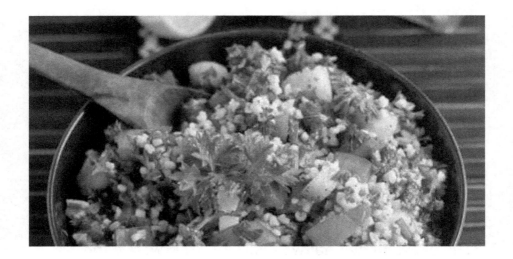

Stuffed Poblano Peppers

Preparation time: 20 minutes
Cooking time: 30 minutes
Servings: 5

Ingredients:

46 g Poblano peppers
2 cups of water
1 cup quinoa
3 tbsp olive oil
1diced onion
2 diced ribs celery
2 diced carrots
2minced garlic cloves
½ cup diced red peppers roasted
1 tbsp adobo sauce with chipotle
2 cup peas
1/3 cup chopped pecans

Directions:

1.Heat the oven before 375°F.

2.With stem, slit each pepper lengthwise. Scoop the seeds out and put them aside.

3Take a medium saucepan, heat water, and add quinoa. Until cooked, boil it and simmer with water immersed. Put it aside.

4.Add olive oil in a medium heated skillet.

5.Sauté the carrots, onion, and celery for about 8 minutes until softened. Then add garlic and for a minute sauté it.

6.Add quinoa cooked before in it and mix well. Add the chipotle, pecans, peas, and roasted red peppers.

7.A shallow baking dish places stuffed peppers and bake them until the peppers are softened for 30 minutes.

8.Serve with meat or a side salad. Enjoy!

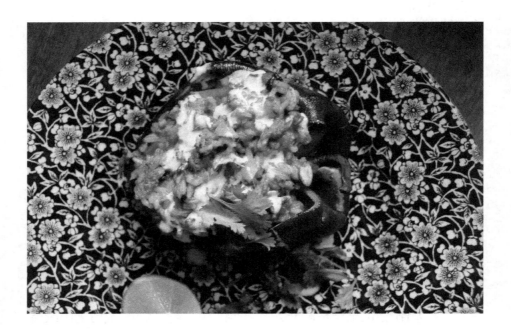

Shiitake, Soba Noodles, and Miso Bowl

Preparation time: 5 minutes
Cooking time: 15 minutes
Servings: 2

Ingredients:

3 cups of water
2 cup dried shiitake mushrooms
4 oz soba noodles
1 tbsp white miso

Directions:

1.In a medium saucepan, boil water over high heat.

2.Add mushrooms and cook them for 6 minutes until swollen and softened.

3.Add in the noodles and cook until al dente.

4.Measure one by 4 cups of noodle broth.

5.Add the miso to it and mix thoroughly with a fork or whisk.

6.Pour this mixture back into the saucepan. Serve in bowls. Enjoy!

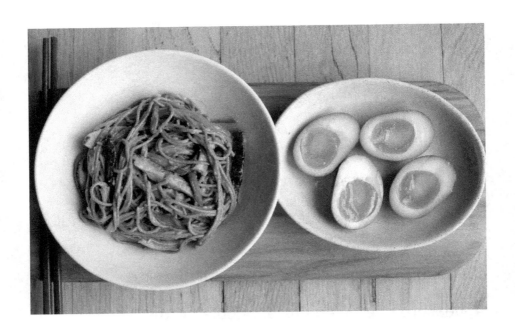

Collard and Rice Stuffed Red Peppers

Preparation time: 10 minutes
Cooking time: 50 minutes
Servings: 4

Ingredients:

2 red bell peppers
2 tbsp olive oil
Black pepper to taste
6 cups collard greens
½ chopped sweet onion
3 minced garlic cloves
1 cup of white rice cooked
2 tbsp lemon Juice
¼ cup roasted sunflower seeds

Directions:

1.Preheat oven at 400°F.

2.Cut half the peppers and remove the stems and seeds. Brush the inside and out with one tbsp of olive oil. Spice them with pepper and put the baking dish cut side down.

3.Until just tender, bake them for ten to fifteen minutes. Flip-up the cut- side of peppers after removing them from the oven and leave the oven on.

4.Take a large saucepan and boil four cups of water. Cook collard greens in it until just tender, for about five to seven minutes. Drain and rinse them under cold water. Then Chop them finely.

63

5.Take a large skillet, and at medium heat, put the left behind tbsp of olive oil. Add in the onion, stir and cook for five to seven minutes, until it turns brown. Add in and cook garlic until it is fragrant.

6.Mix in the collard greens. Put it off from the stove, and add rice and lemon juice in it. Spice it up with pepper.

7.Divide this filling into the pepper halves and crest each half with one tbsp of sunflower seeds. Add one by the fourth cup of water in a baking dish, wrap it with aluminum foil. Bake it for twenty minutes, until it is heated through. Uncover it and then bake again for five more minutes.

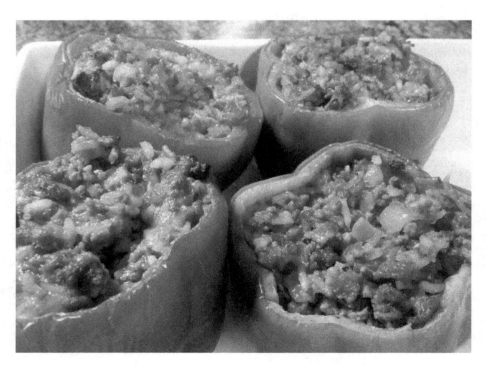

Ginger yogurt dresses the citrus salad

Preparation time: 15 minutes
Cooking time: 0 minute
Servings: 6

Ingrediets:

1.grapefruit Two tangerines 2/3 cup ginger
1/4 cup sugar
2 tbsp honey
3 navel oranges
1/2 cup cranberries
1/4 tsp cinnamon
17.6 oz Greek yogurt

Directions:

1.Break the grapefruit.

2.Cut grapefruit threads, cut the tangerine sections into half.

3.Transfer the grapefruit, all juices & tangerines into a deep serving bowl.

4.Use a small sharp knife,

5.Slice oranges into round shapes and slices into quarters.

6.Add oranges & all juices into a bowl. Mix in cranberries, cinnamon & honey.

7.Cover & refrigerate for 1 hour.

8.Then Mix yogurt & ginger in a bowl.

9.Sprinkle brown sugar & cranberries.

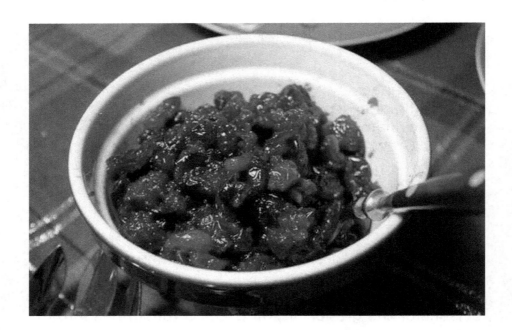

Grilled halloumi cheese salad

Preparation time: 10 minutes
Cooking time: 5 minutes
Servings: 4

Ingredients:
Salad
8 oz Halloumi cheese
1 cup black olives
1/2 cup green olives
2 cups tomatoes
4 cups arugula
1 tbsp olive oil
4 cups shishito peppers
1 cup mint

1/2 cup chives Honey Citrus Dressing

One garlic cloves

1 tsp Dijon mustard
2 tsp honey
2 tsp lemon juice
1/4 cup olive oil
Salt and pepper
1 tsp thyme optional Chili optional

Directions:

1.Cut down the cheese into 0.5-inch slices and soak them in water if required.

2.Heat the grill pan & then adds olive oil to it.

3.Take the cheese slices and grill every slice for 1 to 2 minutes, from one side.

4.Remove the cheese, add the peppers, & increase the temp.

5.Let the peppers cook for three minutes per side.

6.Let the peppers cool down & then chop them with the cheese into small cubes.

7.Mix these with the remaining salad items.

8.Transfer everything in a small bowl and Enjoy

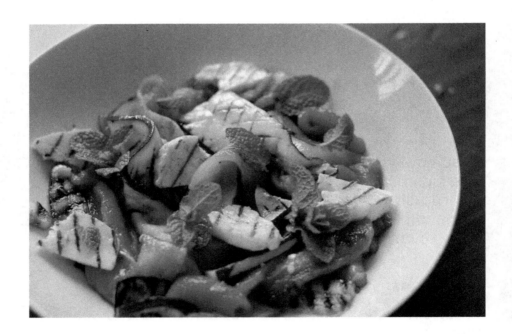

Herbed calamari salad

Preparation time: 20 minutes
Cooking time: 5 minutes
Servings: 6

Ingredients:

3 tbsp extra virgin olive oil
2 minced garlic cloves
2.5 lb calamari rings
1/4 cup cilantro leaves
1/2 cup leaf parsley leaves
3/4 tsp kosher salt
1/4 tsp black pepper
1 pinch of red pepper juice of one lemon
1/4 cup mint leaves Sliced peel of one lemon

Directions:

1.Defrost the calamari. With the help of a cutting, the knife removes skin from the preserved lemon. Remove the inside portion & Slice them into thin pieces.

2.Chop garlic & mince also chop washed parsley, cilantro, & mint.

3.Heat frying pan at high temperature and the add 1.5tbsp. of olive oil to it

4.Heat oil again and add garlic to it and cook with continuous stirring for 20-30 sec. Cook until it is scented, then add calamari batches in it. Divide the 1.5 tbsp. Olive oil in it and cook the calamari batches.

5.Add a pinch of Black pepper & sea salt & continue cooking for 2 to 4 minutes. Or cook until it becomes opaque & firm. Do not overcook it otherwise;, it becomes a rubber-like mixture.

6.Remove the excess liquid left during cooking and convert the coked calamari into a mixing bowl.

7.Add remaining pepper, olive oil, salt, red pepper, preserved lemon rind, herbs, & lemon juice in a mixing bowl & cook well while calamari still warm.

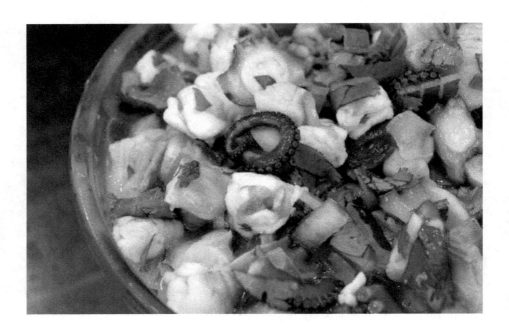

Spring soup with a poached egg

Preparation time: 20 minutes
Cooking time: 20 minutes
Servings: 6

Ingredients:

3 tbsp Olive Oil
2 Leeks
6 Eggs
2 tbsp splash Vinegar
3 Carrots
6 cups Chicken Stock
1 bunch Asparagus
1 bunch Ramps root
2 Garlic cloves
1/2 Sugar Snap Peas
1/2 Mixed Herbs
Lemon Juice

Directions:

1.Heat olive oil in a soup pot, then add carrots, leeks, garlic, and the diced ramp stalks. Flavor with salt & cook on over -high temp. Unless it softens, & the garlic starts to turn golden about 5 minutes.

2.Add the stock and bring to a boil, then reduce to a simmer. Simmer until the vegetables are tender, about 10 minutes.

3.Add the asparagus & pea pods & continue to simmer until the asparagus & peas are crisp-tender, about three mints.

4.Add a pinch of salt & a splash of vinegar. Crack an egg into a cup &

5.gently lower into the simmering water. Turn off the heat, cover the frypan, & let the eggs poach for 4 minutes.

6.Remove eggs & place one egg in the bottom of every soup bowl.

7.Finally, remove from stove & mix the ramp herbs & leaves.

8.Taste & season as needed with sea salt, pepper, & lemon juice.

9.Serve & enjoy your soup.

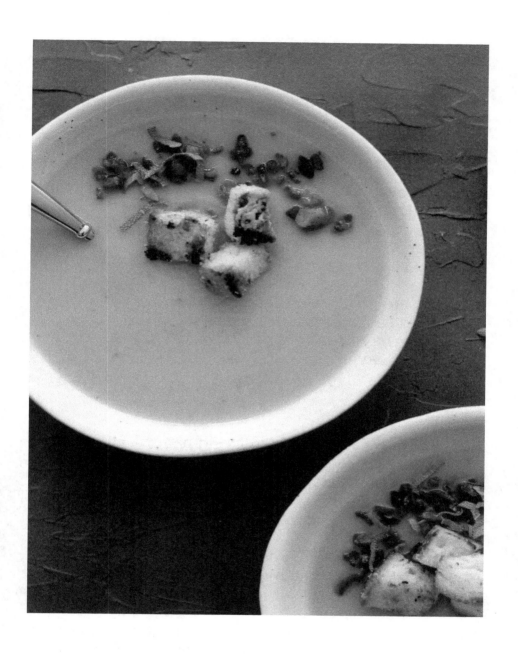

Cucumber olive rice

Preparation time: 30 minutes
Cooking time: 55 minutes
Servings: 8

Iingredients:

3 garlic cloves
1 lb. heirloom
8 oz feta
1 cup parsley leaves
7 tbsp olive oil Kosher
Salt to taste Black pepper to taste
1.5 cups brown rice One chopped onion
3 chopped cucumbers
3 tbsp sherry vinegar
1 cup mint leaves

Directions:

1.Add 2 tbsp. Oil in a heated frying pan.

2.Then add garlic along with salt and cook it for five minutes. While stirring till it gives aroma & transparent. Transfer this into a bowl

3.Take frying pan again, heat it and add 1 tbsp of oil & rice. Cook this for three minutes while stirring till it turns golden & nutty.

4.Add water to the bowl and boil it. Mix it only one time & then decrease the heat to low temp. and then cover it. Cook till rice is delicate, & water has been soaked up.

5.Please remove it from the stove and let it cool for five minutes.
6.Move rice into a bowl along with the mixture of onion and let it cool for 20 minutes.

7.Mix cucumbers, tomatoes, vinegar, & remaining oil. Season with sea salt & black pepper.

8.Finally, Coat with cheese, parsley, & mint and serve it.

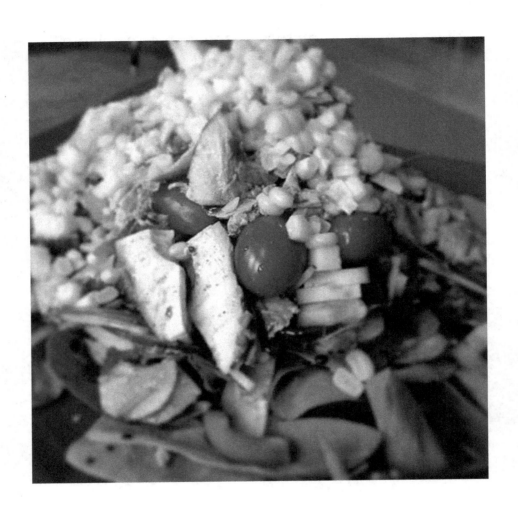

Basil tomato rice

Preparation time: 10 minutes
Cooking time: 30 minutes
Servings: 4

Ingredints:

1 tbsp olive oil
2 cloves garlic
Salt to taste
Black pepper to taste
1/2 cup onion
1 cup white rice
1 ripe tomato
2 cups chicken broth
3 tbsp grated parmesan cheese
2 tbsp basil

Directions:

1.Take a frying pan, add onions & olive oil to it and cook it for four minutes. Then add rice in it & cook it for 2-3 mints more.

2.Add tomatoes, chicken broth, sale, black pepper & garlic to it.

3.Cover it and boil & reduce heat to a simmer. Cook for 20 minutes. Without raising the lid.

4Please remove it from the stove & rest it for five minutes before removing the lid off. Add parmesan cheese & basil & mix well.

5.Place this in a bowl and garnish it with remaining parmesan cheese along with basil & tomatoes if required.

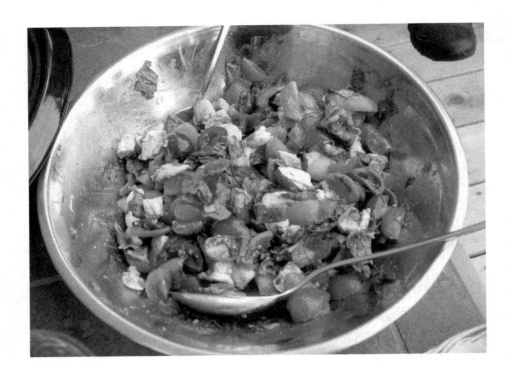

Watermelon Bowl

Preparation Time: 1 hour and 10 minutes
Cooking Time: 0 minutes
Servings: 32

Ingredients:

1 Watermelon, Halved Lengthwise
3 Tablespoons Lime Juice, Fresh
1 Cup Sugar
1 ½ Cup Water
1 ½ Cups Mint Leaves, Fresh & Chopped
6 Plums, Pitted & Halved
1 Cantaloupe, Small
4 Nectarines, Pitted & Halved
1 lb. Green Grapes, Seedless

Directions:

1.Mix sugar and water in a two-quart pot and bring it to a boil using medium heat. Stir your sugar in until it dissolves.

2.Mix in your lime juice and mint, and then place it in the fridge until chilled. Chop your watermelon and cantaloupe into bite sized pieces, and then slice the nectarines and plums into wedges.

3.Mix all your fruit in a large bowl before adding in your grapes. Take the mixture out of the fridge and pour it over the fruit.
Mix well, and then cover it with saran wrap.

4.Refrigerate for two hours, and stir occasionally. Serve chilled.

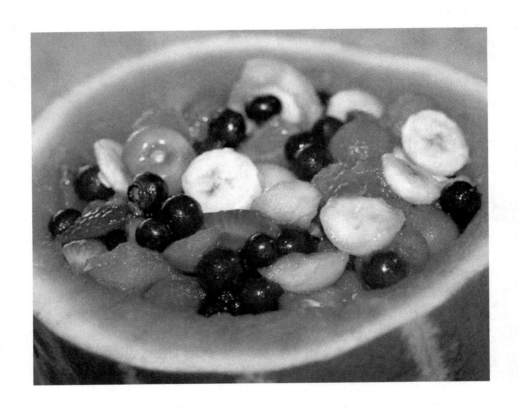

Red Egg Skillet

Preparation Time: 5 minutes
Cooking Time: 10 minutes
Servings: 6

Ingredients:

7 Greek Olives, Pitted & Sliced
3 Tomatoes, Ripe & Diced
2 Tablespoons Olive oil
4 Eggs
¼ Cup Parsley, Fresh & Chopped
1/8 Teaspoon Sea Salt,
Fine Black Pepper to Taste

Directions:

1. Get out a pan and grease it. Throw your tomatoes in and cook for ten minutes before adding in your olives. Cook for another five minutes.

2. Add your eggs into the pan, cooking over medium-heat so that your eggs are cooked all the way through.

3. Season with salt and pepper and serve topped with parsley.

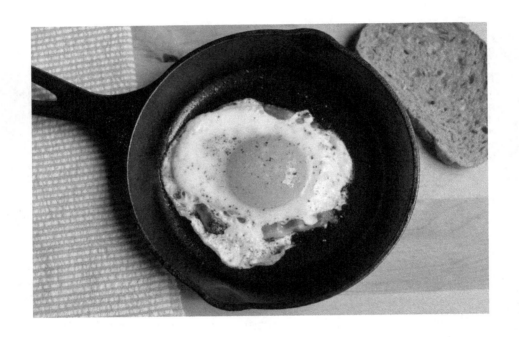

Roasted Plum with Almonds

Preparation Time: 15 minutes
Cooking Time: 30 minutes
Servings: 6
Ingredients:

6 Plums, Large, Pitted & Halved
3 Tablespoons butter
1/3 Cup Brown Sugar
2 Cups Fennel, Sliced
¼ Cup All Purpose Flour
1/3 Cup Almonds, Sliced

Directions:

1.Heat your oven to 425, and then place the plums in a shallow baking dish.

2.Get out a shallow baking dish and place your plums inside.
Get out a bowl, mix your brown sugar and butter until smooth, and blend in your flour. Make sure it's mixed well, and then toss in your almonds.

3.Pour the mixture over the plums evenly, and then bake for twenty-five to thirty minutes. The plums should be tender.

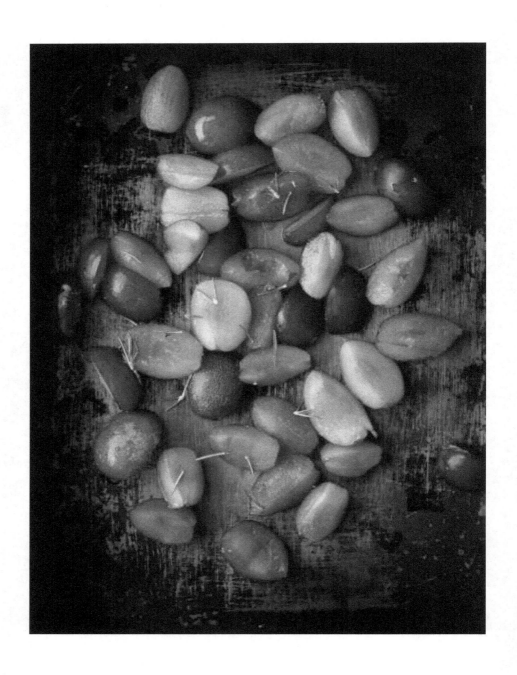

Cappuccino Muffins

Preparation Time: 10 minutes
Cooking Time: 25 minutes
Servings: 12

Ingredients:

2 Cups Flour, All Purpose
1 Egg
½ Cup Cream
1 Tablespoon Baking Powder
1/8 Teaspoon Sea Salt, Fine
½ Cup Brown Sugar
1 Cup Coffee, Cold
Powdered Sugar for Garnish

Directions:

1.Start by heating your oven to 350, and then grease a muffin tray using butter. Sift your salt, baking powder and flour together in a bowl.

2.Beat your eggs along with your cream together until it's blended well. Pour this mixture in a floured bowl, and mix well.

3.Stir in your coffee, and then divide between your muffin tins. Bake for twenty minutes, and serve garnished with powder sugar.

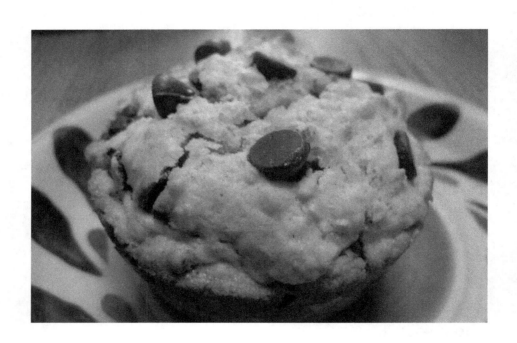

Cooked Beef Mushroom Egg

Preparation Time: 10 minutes
Cooking Time: 15 minutes
Servings: 2

Ingredients:

¼ cup cooked beef, diced
6 eggs
3 mushrooms, diced
Salt and pepper to taste
12 ounces spinach
2 onions, chopped
A dash of onion powder
¼ green bell pepper, chopped
A dash of garlic powder

Directions:

1.In a skillet, toss the beef for 3 minutes or until crispy. Take off the heat and add to a plate.

2.Add the onion, bell pepper, and mushroom in the skillet. Add the rest of the ingredients.

3.Toss for about 4 minutes.

4.Return the beef to the skillet and toss for another minute. Serve hot.

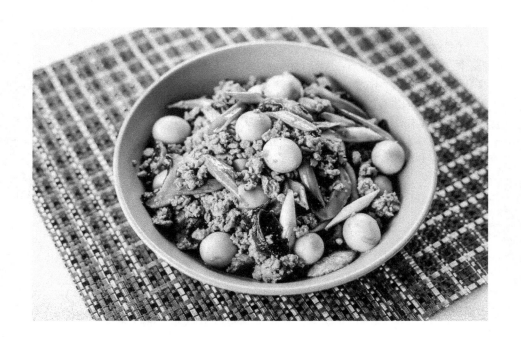

Curried Veggies and Poached Eggs

Preparation Time: 20 minutes
Cooking Time: 45 minutes
Servings: 4

Ingredients:

4 large eggs
½ tsp. white vinegar
1/8 tsp. crushed red pepper – optional
1 cup water
1 14-oz. can chickpeas, drained
2 medium zucchinis, diced
½ lb. sliced button mushrooms
1 tbsp. yellow curry powder
2 cloves garlic, minced
1 large onion, chopped
2 tsp.s. extra virgin olive oil

Directions:

1.On medium high fire, place a large saucepan and heat oil. Sauté onions until tender around four to five minutes.

2.Add garlic and continue sautéing for another half minute.
Add curry powder, stir and cook until fragrant around one to two minutes.

3.Add mushrooms, mix, cover and cook for 5 to 8 minutes or until mushrooms are tender and have released their liquid.

4.Add red pepper if using, water, chickpeas and zucchini. Mix well to combine and bring to a boil.

5.Once boiling, reduce fire to a simmer, cover and cook until zucchini is tender around 15 to 20 minutes of simmering.
6.Meanwhile, in a small pot filled with 3-inches deep water, bring to a boil on high fire.

7.Once boiling, reduce fire to a simmer and add vinegar.
Slowly add one egg, slipping it gently into the water. Allow to simmer until egg is cooked, around 3 to 5 minutes.

8.Remove egg with a slotted spoon and transfer to a plate, one plate one egg. Repeat the process with remaining eggs.

9.Once the veggies are done cooking, divide evenly into 4 servings and place one serving per egg plate.
Serve and enjoy.

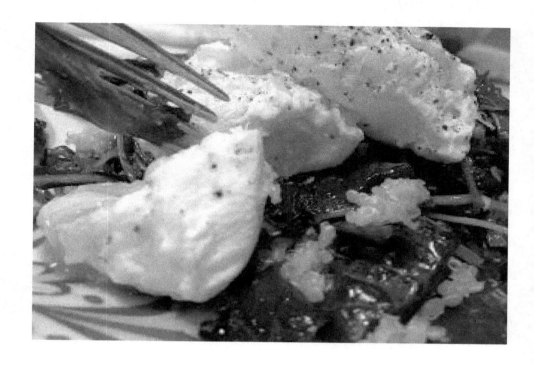

Eggs over Kale Hash

Preparation Time: 10 minutes
Cooking Time: 20 minutes
Servings: 4

Ingredients:

4 large eggs
1 bunch chopped kale
Dash of ground nutmeg
2 sweet potatoes, cubed
1 14.5-ounce can of chicken broth

Directions:

1.In a large non-stick skillet, bring the chicken broth to a simmer. Add the sweet potatoes and season slightly with salt and pepper.

2.Add a dash of nutmeg to improve the flavor. Cook until the sweet potatoes become soft, around 10 minutes. Add kale and season with salt and pepper. Continue cooking for four minutes or until kale has wilted. Set aside.

3.Using the same skillet, heat 1 tablespoon of olive oil over medium high heat. Cook the eggs sunny side up until the whites become opaque and the yolks have set.

4.Top the kale hash with the eggs. Serve immediately.

Italian Scrambled Eggs

Preparation Time: 10 minutes
Cooking Time: 7 minutes
Servings: 1

Ingredients:

1 teaspoon balsamic vinegar
2 large eggs
¼ teaspoon rosemary, minced
½ cup cherry tomatoes
1 ½ cup kale, chopped
½ teaspoon olive oil

Directions:

1.Melt the olive oil in a skillet over medium high heat. Sauté the kale and add rosemary and salt to taste. Add three tablespoons of water to prevent the kale from burning at the bottom of the pan. Cook for three to four minutes.

2.Add the tomatoes and stir.

3.Push the vegetables on one side of the skillet and add the eggs. Season with salt and pepper to taste. Scramble the eggs then fold in the tomatoes and kales.

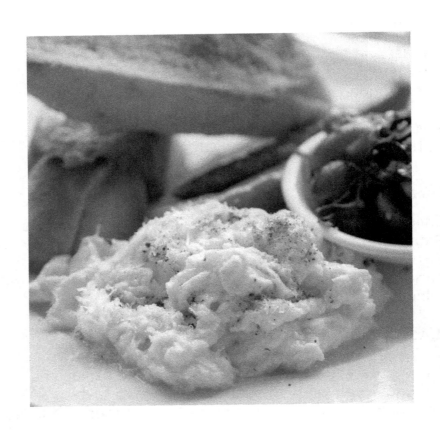

Lettuce Stuffed with Eggs 'n Crab Meat

Preparation Time: 15 minutes
Cooking Time: 10 minutes
Servings: 8

Ingredients:

24 butter lettuce leaves
1 tsp. dry mustard
¼ cup finely chopped celery
1 cup lump crabmeat, around 5 ounces
3 tbsp. plain Greek yogurt
2 tbsp. extra virgin olive oil
¼ tsp. ground pepper
8 large eggs
½ tsp. salt, divided
1 tbsp. fresh lemon juice, divided
2 cups thinly sliced radishes

Directions:

1.In a medium bowl, mix ¼ tsp. salt, 2 tsp.s. Juice and radishes. Cover and chill for half an hour.

2.On medium saucepan, place eggs and cover with water over an inch above the eggs. Bring the pan of water to a boil. Once boiling, reduce fire to a simmer and cook for ten minutes.

3.Turn off fire, discard hot water and place eggs in an ice water bath to cool completely.
Peel eggshells and slice eggs in half lengthwise and remove the yolks.

4.With a sieve on top of a bowl, place yolks and press through a sieve. Set aside a tablespoon of yolk.
On remaining bowl of yolks add pepper, ¼ tsp. salt and 1 tsp. juice.

5.Mix well and as you are stirring, slowly add oil until well incorporated. Add yogurt, stir well to mix.

6.Add mustard, celery and crabmeat. Gently mix to combine. If needed, taste and adjust seasoning of the filling.

7.On a serving platter, arrange 3 lettuce in a fan for two egg slices. To make the egg whites sit flat, you can slice a bit of the bottom to make it flat. Evenly divide crab filling into egg white holes.

8.Then evenly divide into eight servings the radish salad and add on the eggs' side, on top of the lettuce leaves. Serve and enjoy.

Parmesan and Poached Eggs on Asparagus

Preparation Time: 10 minutes
Cooking Time: 15 minutes
Servings: 4

Ingredients:

4 tbsp. coarsely grated fresh Parmesan cheese, divided
Freshly ground black pepper, to taste
2 tsp.s. finely chopped fresh parsley
2 tbsp. fresh lemon juice
1 tbsp. unsalted butter
1 garlic clove, chopped
1 tbsp. extra virgin olive oil
2 bunches asparagus spears, trimmed around 40
1 tsp. salt, divided
1 tsp. white vinegar
8 large eggs

Directions:

1.Break eggs and place in one paper cup per egg. On medium high fire, place a low sided pan filled 3/4 with water. Add ½ tsp. salt and vinegar into water. Set aside.

2.On medium high fire bring another pot of water to boil. Once boiling, lower fire to a simmer and blanch asparagus until tender and crisp, around 3-4 minutes. With tongs transfer asparagus to a serving platter and set aside.

3.On medium fire, place a medium saucepan and heat olive oil. Once hot, for a minute sauté garlic and turn off fire. Add butter right away and swirl around pan to melt. Add remaining pepper, salt, parsley and lemon juice and mix thoroughly.

4.Add asparagus and toss to combine well with garlic butter sauce. Transfer to serving platter along with sauce.

5.In boiling pan of water, poach the eggs by pouring eggs into the water slowly and cook for two minutes per egg.

6.With a slotted spoon, remove egg, remove excess water, tap slotted spoon several times on kitchen towel, and place it on top of asparagus.

7.To serve, top eggs with parmesan cheese and divide the asparagus into two and 2 eggs per plate. Serve and enjoy.

Scrambled eggs with Smoked Salmon

Preparation Time: 15 minutes
Cooking Time: 8 minutes
Servings: 1

Ingredients:

1 tbsp. coconut oil Pepper and salt to taste
1/8 tsp. red pepper flakes
1/8 tsp. garlic powder
1 tbsp. fresh dill, chopped finely
4 oz. smoked salmon, torn apart
2 whole eggs + 1 egg yolk, whisked

Directions:

1.In a big bowl whisk the eggs. Mix in pepper, salt, red pepper flakes, garlic, dill and salmon.

2.On low fire, place a nonstick fry pan and lightly grease with oil.
Pour egg mixture and whisk around until cooked through to make scrambled eggs, around 8 minutes on medium fire.

3.Serve and enjoy.

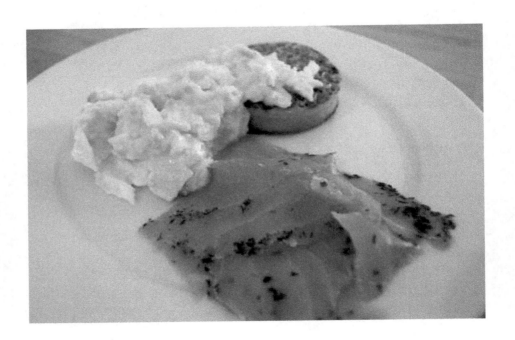

Scrambled Eggs with Feta 'n Mushrooms

Preparation Time: 5 minutes
Cooking Time: 6 minutes
Servings: 1

Ingredients:

Pepper to taste
2 tbsp. feta cheese
1 whole egg
2 egg whites
1 cup fresh spinach, chopped
½ cup fresh mushrooms, sliced
Cooking spray

Directions:

1.On medium high fire, place a nonstick fry pan and grease with cooking spray. Once hot, add spinach and mushrooms.

2.Sauté until spinach is wilted, around 2-3 minutes. Meanwhile, in a bowl whisk well egg, egg whites, and cheese. Season with pepper.

3.Pour egg mixture into pan and scramble until eggs are cooked through, around 3-4 minutes.

4.Serve and enjoy with a piece of toast or brown rice.

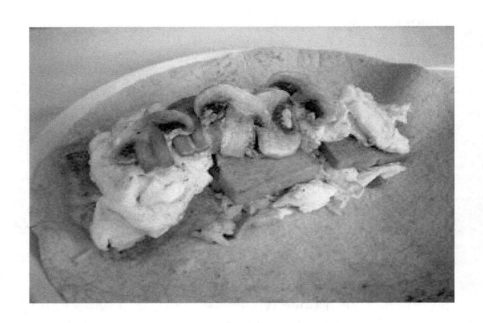

Belly-Filling Cajun Rice & Chicken

Preparation Time: 15 minutes
Cooking Time: 20 minutes
Servings: 6

Ingredients:

1 tablespoon oil
1 onion, diced
3 cloves of garlic, minced
1-pound chicken breasts, sliced
1 tablespoon Cajun seasoning
1 tablespoon tomato paste
2 cups chicken broth
1 ½ cups white rice, rinsed
1 bell pepper, chopped

Directions:

1.Press the Sauté on the Instant Pot and pour the oil. Sauté the onion and garlic until fragrant.

2.Stir in the chicken breasts and season with Cajun seasoning. Continue cooking for 3 minutes.

3.Add the tomato paste and chicken broth. Dissolve the tomato paste before adding the rice and bell pepper.

4.Close the lid and press the rice button.
Once done cooking, do a natural release for 10 minutes. Then, do a quick release.

5.Once cooled, evenly divide into serving size, keep in your preferred container, and refrigerate until ready to eat.

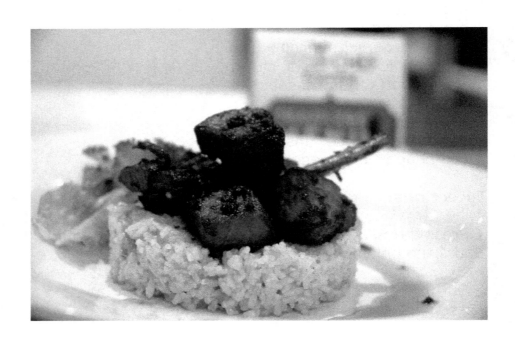

The Bell Pepper Fiesta

Preparation Time: 10 minutes
Cooking Time: 0 minutes
Servings: 4

Ingredients:

1 tablespoons dill, chopped
1 yellow onion, chopped
1 pound multi colored peppers, cut, halved, seeded and cut into thin strips
1 tbsp organic olive oil
½ tablespoons white wine vinegar
Black pepper to taste

Directions:

1.Take a bowl and mix in sweet pepper, onion, dill, pepper, oil, vinegar and toss well.

2.Divide between bowls and serve.

3.Enjoy!

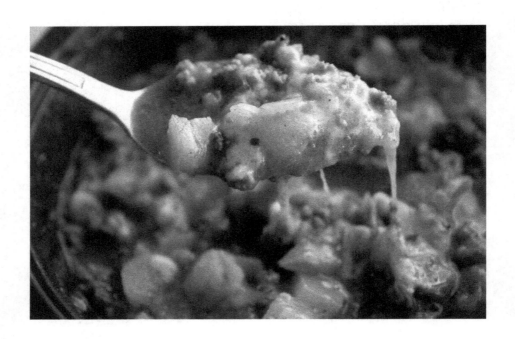

Spiced Up Pumpkin Seeds Bowls

Preparation Time: 10 minutes
Cooking Time: 20 minutes
Servings: 4

Ingredients:

½ tablespoon chili powder
½ teaspoon cayenne
1 cups pumpkin seeds
teaspoons lime juice

Directions:

1.Spread pumpkin seeds over lined baking sheet; add lime juice, cayenne and chili powder.

2.Toss well.

3.Pre-heat your oven to 275 degrees F.

4.Roast in your oven for 20 minutes and transfer to small bowls.

5.Serve and enjoy!

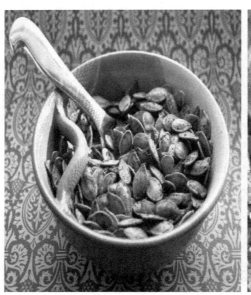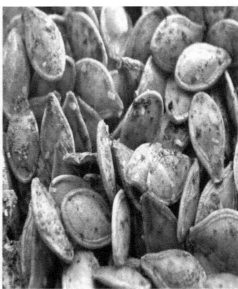

Chicken Salad

Preparation Time: 5 Minutes
Cooking Time: 30 Minutes
Servings: 2

Ingredients:

½ red onion, very finely sliced
1 tablespoon of sesame seeds
150g of cooked chicken-shredded
Large handful 20g of parsley-chopped
100g of baby kale-chopped roughly
1 teaspoons of soy sauce
1 teaspoon of clear honey
1 teaspoon of sesame oil

Directions:

1. Place a frying pan over medium heat.

2.Mix the sesame oil, honey, olive oil, lime juice, and soy sauce to make the dressing.

3.Place the cucumber, red onion, kale, pak choi, and parsley in a large bowl and gently mix.

4.Pour the dressing over and mix again.

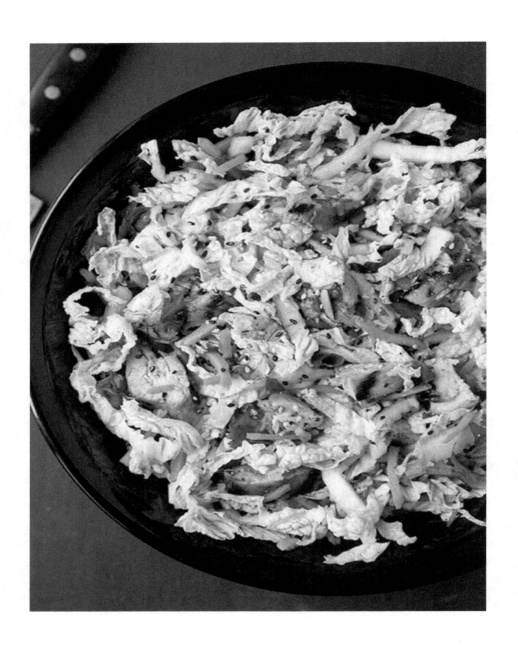

9 781802 690224